The Lymphoedema Diet:

reverse and repair lymphatic damage

By
Lynne D M Noble

Copyright 2019 Lynne D M Noble

Independently published

About the Author

Lynne Noble was born in 1953 in Huddersfield, West Yorkshire. From a very early age, Lynne showed an interest in nutrition and genetics avidly reading any books that she could get her hands on at the time.

Initially, Lynne studied orthopaedics but events led her to work with the elderly mentally infirm. Here, her interest in neurodegenerative disorders and pain syndromes developed.

Lynne undertook rigorous programmes of study, completing her Cert Ed., (FE) BSc (Hons) and Adv. Dip Education simultaneously before moving onto her M.Ed.

From there she took further demanding programmes in Human Nutrition, Pharmacology, Neuroscience, Genetics and Immunology. During this time, she was given many prestigious awards for her academic work. It was noted then that Lynne was not afraid of tackling difficult subjects.

She began her law degree but ill health prevented her from pursuing this. However, in this time, she moved from being a foster parent to adoptive parent.

She has been instrumental in setting up projects in the community for disadvantaged groups.

She is a member of the Guild of Health Writers.

Now retired, she lives in a picturesque village in West Yorkshire with her husband. She enjoys gardening, watching her husband bowling and researching.

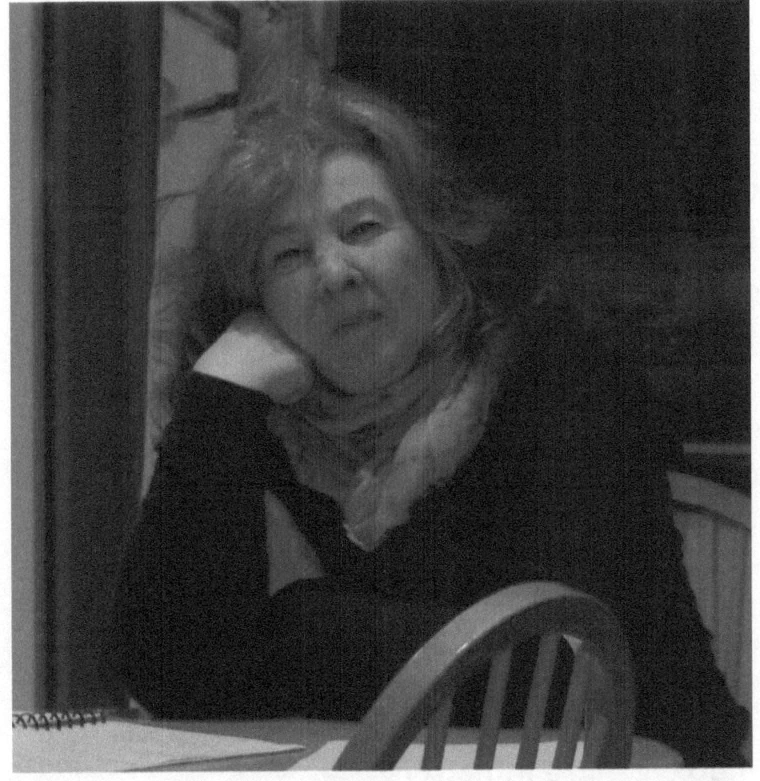

Author Lynne Noble at home

https://quintessentiallylynne.weebly.com/nutritional-medicine.html

Contents

Preface

Lymphoedema is a chronic disease which can cause unsightly swelling in any part of the body due to a damaged lymphatic system.

The symptoms of lymphoedema are increasing disability, disfigurement and pain. The current treatments the wearing of compression garments 24 hours, in addition to a technique known as manual lymphatic drainage. This assists the passage of stagnant lymph to move through the system. Nevertheless, these treatments do not address the underlying processes of lymphoedema which carries with it a high risk of infection.

Lymphoedema generally occurs after surgery or during cancer therapy treatment; sometimes the manifestation of lymphoedema may occur immediately after the event. However, in some cases, it can manifest itself years later.

Once thought to be irreversible and due to a plumbing problem, a ground breaking study has now uncovered the molecular mechanism responsible for triggering lymphoedema. Lymphoedema is now known to be due to inflammation – not a plumbing problem.

The underlying inflammatory nature of lymphoedema was discovered when studies showed that ketoprofen – an anti-inflammatory substance - was successful in alleviating the symptoms of lymphoedema.

While a drug - to reverse the chronic inflammation underpinning lymphoedema - is still in the offing, there are a number of nutritional substances which can inhibit the inflammatory processes that are known to help develop and progress lymphoedema. These nutritional substances address the pathological pathways found in lymphoedema. They help reduce and reverse the damaging effects of inflammation and microvascular permeability.

This book is intended to inform lymphoedema patients of the latest research about this condition. In addition, it shows how nutritional substances can assist in inhibiting or progressing this condition.

While there is a little chemistry involved, I have – where I thought it judicious – to include further explanations, so that all readers may benefit from what the latest findings have to offer for those with lymphoedema.

What is lymphoedema?

The NHS[1] describes lymphoedema as:

'a long term (chronic) condition that causes swelling in the body's tissues. It can affect any part of the body, but usually develops in the arms or legs. It develops when the lymphatic system doesn't work properly.'

The lymphatic system consists of a network of canals and glands that can be found throughout the body. It has two main functions:

- Fighting infection
- Removing any excess fluid

Primary lymphoedema is due to faulty genes and starts in childhood. It is not as common as secondary lymphoedema which generally occurs due to infection, injury, lack of limb movement, obesity, cancer treatment and varicose veins. Up until recently, this list would include 'and inflammation in the limb.' Now we

---

[1]

https://www.nhs.uk/conditions/lymphoedema/

know that lymphoedema *is* inflammation in the limb – chronic inflammation; that is, inflammation that serves no useful purpose.

Somewhere during the initial development of lymphoedema, an infection or injury has occurred. When infection or injury occurs, acute inflammatory processes spring into gear to repair the damage. This is to be expected and is not a pathological process at this stage.

We would expect the inflammatory processes to stop once complete healing has taken place. In some cases, this does not happen. Acute inflammation progresses to chronic inflammation. Chronic inflammation serves no useful purpose whatsoever. It does not allow healing to take place. Instead, the chronic inflammatory processes begin to destroy tissue.

Varicose veins as a risk factor for lymphoedema

Varicose veins are a risk factor for lymphoedema.

Varicose veins are swollen or enlarged veins and normally – but not confined to – the legs. They develop when blood does not flow through the veins well, due to incompetent valves. This causes high vein pressure. Subsequently, fluid overflows into the surrounding tissues.

Studies[2] have shown that leg samples from patients with varicose veins had significantly higher levels of IL-6, IL-8 and MCP-1 compared to their own arm samples. These are markers of inflammation. We shall look at these immune system markers, shortly.

Varicose veins may need to be removed so that blood will be shunted to veins which are working well and would be able to deal with the flow of blood. This would prevent excess fluid from leaking into surrounding tissues.

Unfortunately, the removal of varicose veins is often seen as a cosmetic treatment making it unavailable to many who would benefit from it.

---

[2] https://www.ncbi.nlm.nih.gov/pubmed/27103338

However, it is advised to ask for a referral to a vascular consultant if varicose veins are troublesome and may be contributing to lymphoedema. While most are visible, it is still possible to have varicose veins, that lie much deeper within the tissue and they can just be as problematical as the more superficial ones.

The immune system markers found in varicose veins

AMP-1. These are antimicrobial peptides[3] that are also known as host defense peptides (HDP's) and are part of the innate immune system[4]. They can kill Gram negative and Gram positive bacteria, enveloped viruses, fungi and mutated or cancerous cells. Their presence suggests that an infective agent may be somehow involved in the development and/or maintenance of varicose veins.

---

[3] Tiny particles of protein that fight infection

[4] The innate immune system is the infection fighting system that you are born with as opposed to the acquired immune system which develops as you are exposed to infection.

Interleukin-8 is a cytokine. This means it is secreted from cells of the immune system and affects other cells. In IL-8's case it mainly attracts and activates neutrophils in inflammatory regions. Neutrophils are a type of white blood cell that helps to heal damaged tissues and resolve infections.

IL-6 – This cytokine is secreted by T cells and macrophages to activate immune responses during infection or after trauma.

The presence of AMP-1, IL-6 and IL-8, in veins, suggests the existence of a low grade infection or damage to the endothelial cells lining the veins.

Infection or injury will result in inflammatory processes which may develop into a chronic condition such as lymphoedema.

The role of obesity in lymphoedema

Weight reduction is recommended as one of a number of treatments for lymphoedema. The development of varicose veins is said to progress more rapidly in overweight people. This may not be the whole story. There are individuals who are not overweight who have a predisposition to varicose veins and overweight people who do not succumb to them. Nevertheless, exercise helps increase lymph flow which becomes sluggish and stagnant in lymphoedema, increasing the risk for infection. Exercise also encourages deeper breathing. This helps the deeper lymphatic channels in the abdomen to drain.

And just like varicose veins, obesity is also considered to be an inflammatory condition.

This is a fairly simple overview of some of the more prevalent conditions - often found alongside lymphoedema - that are also linked to chronic inflammation. Of course, up until recently, lymphoedema was thought to be due to a plumbing problem. Now we know it is not. As such, this appears to be a suitable place to stop and move onto the ground breaking study that has demonstrated that lymphoedema is not due to a plumbing problem but is a condition that occurs due to the presence of chronic inflammation.

The study

The study that revealed that lymphoedema was a condition of inflammation - and not one due to a 'plumbing' problem - was undertaken by[5] a Petit Institute researcher, Brandon Dixon. It considered to be a ground breaking study. The study was published on May 10th 2018 in *Science Translational Medicine.*

The researchers found that an inflammatory substance called leukotriene B4 (also known as LTB4) was elevated in both animal models and humans with lymphoedema.

When LTB4 levels are elevated then inflammation of the tissues occurs. This impairs lymphatic function. Leukotrienes have far reaching effects. Some of these are described below.

The negative effects of leukotrienes

---

[5] http://www.rh.gatech.edu/news/591638/first-possible-drug-treatment-lymphedema

Leukotrienes are well known for their negative effects on asthma. Acute asthma attacks are often triggered by exercise or allergens. Leukotrienes are released by mast cells[6] and are involved in bronchoconstriction.

 In addition, they increase mucous secretion in both asthma and chronic obstructive pulmonary disease (COPD). Further, they are implicated in arthritis and atherosclerosis, as well as some cancers.

During inflammatory processes, leukotrienes increase microvascular permeability.

It is the inflammatory processes of leukotrienes that needs to be targeted since it has been identified that it is this that initiates and progresses lymphoedema.

Further research found that when drugs were used that specifically targeted LTB4 then lymphatic repair was instigated and the disease process, and damage, was eventually reversed.

---

[6] Mast cells are responsible for allergic reactions

A researcher, Tian, in this study, stated.

'There is currently no drug treatment for lymphedema. Based on results of the study the drug bestatin, which is not approved for use in the United States but which has been used for decades in Japan to treat cancer, was found to work well as an LTB4 inhibitor, with no side effects.'

This insight is good news since there are many nutrients which can also inhibit LTB4. However, first it may be helpful to examine what leukotrienes actually are.

Leukotrienes, arachidonic acid and omega 6 PUFA's

The biochemical definition is:

Any of a group of biologically active compounds, originally isolated from leucocytes (white blood cells). They are metabolites of arachidonic acid, containing three conjugated bonds.

That's a bit of a mouthful so let's pull it apart and see what it really means.

A **leucocyte** is simply a white blood cell. They protect the body against infectious disease and foreign invaders.

A **metabolite** is the very end product of some chemical processes, that occur in a living organism, in order to maintain life.

Leukotrienes are the end product of **arachidonic acid.**

Arichidonic acid is a polyunsaturated omega-6 fatty acid. It is found in the membranes of the body's cells and is particularly abundant in the brain, muscles and liver. It is a key inflammatory intermediate and can act as a vasodilator. This means it can widen blood vessels.

Arichidonic acid has many beneficial roles in the body. It cannot cause inflammation unless tiny particles, called electrons, try and disrupt the stability of other electrons found in the fat that forms part of the cell membranes.

Arachidonic acid can be metabolised to both anti-inflammatory and pro-inflammatory eicanosoids[7]. It is quite likely that if you suffer from joint pain, bronchoconstriction, microvascular permeability and lymphoedema that arachidonic acid has been converted to a pro-inflammatory compound.

---

[7] An eicosanoid is the end product of a process.

Table 4. Food sources of arachidonic acid (PFA 20:4), listed in descending order by percentages of their contribution to intake, based on data from the National Health and Nutrition Examination Survey 2005-2006

Rank	Food item	Contribution to intake (%)	Cumulative contribution (%)
1	Chicken and chicken mixed dishes	26.9	26.9
2	Eggs and egg mixed dishes	17.8	44.7
3	Beef and beef mixed dishes	7.3	52.0
4	Sausage, franks, bacon, and ribs	6.7	58.7
5	Other fish and fish mixed dishes	5.8	64.5
6	Burgers	4.6	69.1
7	Cold cuts	3.3	72.4
8	Pork and pork mixed dishes	3.1	75.5
9	Mexican mixed dishes	3.1	78.7
10	Pizza	2.8	81.5
11	Turkey and turkey mixed dishes	2.7	84.2
12	Pasta and pasta dishes	2.3	86.5
13	Grain-based desserts	2.0	88.5

Specific foods contributing at least 1% of eicosatetraenoic acid in descending order: shrimp and shrimp mixed dishes, soups, regular cheese.

[8]

https://epi.grants.cancer.gov/diet/foodsources/fatty_acids/table4.html

Eicanosoids are a class of compounds (like leukotrienes and prostaglandins) which are synthesised from poly unsaturated fatty acids (PUFA's) - like arachidonic acid – and that are involved in cellular activity. They are lipid mediators of inflammation.

In fact, a study[9] on lymphoedema in breast cancer patients has supported the connection between raised PUFA's and lymphoedema.

The study demonstrated that breast cancer survivors with lymphoedema had elevated PUFA's, arachidonic acid, fatty acid desaturase enzyme activity indices and EPA in serum phospholipids.

The study concluded that the extent of fatty acid composition might be related to the risk of secondary lymphoedema in breast cancer survivors. If these PUFA's have the potential to be so damaging, which foods are they found in and how easy are they to avoid?

---

[9] https://www.ncbi.nlm.nih.gov/pubmed/27041742

Where are PUFA's found?

 Major sources of Omega 6   PUFA's are vegetable oils like Canola oil, grapeseed oil, corn oil, soybean oil, peanut oil among others.

There are plenty of hidden sources of these PUFA's. They are found in ready meals, granola, crisps, energy bars, flax seeds and soups, to name a few.   They are also found in commercially raised poultry, beef and eggs.

In fact, our consumption of PUFA's has risen dramatically since their introduction. They have now replaced the more stable saturated fats such as lard, dripping and butter that were the mainstay of the UK diet until around the early 1970's when the apparently 'healthy' benefits of polyunsaturated fatty acids were heavily marketed.

However, oils which are rich in poly unsaturated fatty acids generate aldehydes freely. Aldehydes promote cancer, heart disease and dementia. In fact, the World Health Organisation found that aldehyde levels were found to be twenty times higher, than recommended levels, in these oils.

Are poly unsaturated fatty acids responsible for the chronic inflammation found in lymphoedema? It is quite possible given that arachidonic acid is a PUFA, and that its end product is LTB4 – the leukotriene that has been found to be responsible for the chronic inflammation found in lymphoedema. However, this isn't quite the whole story.

In the study on breast cancer and lymphoedema it was found that desaturase enzyme levels were elevated. Exactly what are desaturase enzymes?

Enzymes are protein particles that help speed up a process in the body. There are thousands of processes in the body that require diverse enzymes in order to continue. Without enzymatic activity life would cease to exist.

Desaturase enzymes

Desaturase enzymes can convert fatty acids to either pro-inflammatory or anti-inflammatory products. Inflammation helps us repair and heal. It can be seen that at times of injury or illness then pro-inflammatory substances are required to travel to the site of injury or infection. However, when injury or illness does not exist then the conversion of fatty acids to anti- inflammatory products is the desired outcome.   However, desaturase enzymes require a number of other essential nutrients in order to respond appropriately to the body's status. Without these, things can go awry. For example, inflammation can continue long after the need for it has subsided.

Desaturase enzymes are so important to understanding how inflammatory processes may *not* respond appropriately to specific conditions in the body, that they deserve to be highlighted.

What are desaturase enzymes?

Desaturase enzymes help produce and convert fatty acids to their preferred end product- that is, either anti-inflammatory or proinflammatory mediators. These enzymes cannot carry this task out in isolation. For example,

Delta 5-desaturase requires, niacin, zinc and vitamin C

Delta 6-saturase requires enough magnesium, B6 and zinc to function properly.

Zinc deficiency is rare in the developed world but may happen in someone with a poor diet.

Magnesium deficiency is quite common – more so if diuretics or laxatives are taken. Indeed, a study argued that subclinical magnesium deficiency is a public health crisis.

Those people who do not eat a diet with nuts or wholegrains are likely to be vitamin B6 deficient.

Any one of the above deficiencies can help to progress lymphoedema.

Zinc, magnesium and vitamin B6 (the latter is better taken in a complex of B vitamins) may all supplemented. They can generally be obtained at local supermarkets. If not, then they may be obtained at health stores or online.

The recommended dietary allowances are:

Zinc: 11mg for men, 8mg for women

Magnesium: 500mg

Vitamin B6: 1.5mg for women, 2mg for men

The role of 5-lipoxygenase inhibitors in the treatment of lymphoedema.

5-lipoxygenase (5-LO) is a key enzyme in the synthesis of leukotrienes. Its importance as a therapeutic target cannot be underestimated.

5-LO brings about the first two steps of the transformation of arachidonic acid to leukotrienes.

 However, the only clinically approved inhibitor of 5-lipoxygenase – zileuton – has unacceptable side effects.

There are some naturally occurring 5-lipoxygenase inhibitors. These include:

- Caffeic acid phenpropyl ester (found in bee propolis)
- Diphenlethyl ester*
- Phenylpropyl*
- Hypericum perforatum
- Gamma tocotrienol

- Delta tocopherol
- Gamma tocopherol
- Curcumin
- Erucic acid
- Monoenoic fatty acids
- Pumpkin seeds

We shall look at these – and others - in more detail later.

The starred substances above were found[10] to be significantly greater in inhibitory action than the reference molecules – which also showed 5-lipoxygenase inhibitory action. These comprised: caffeic acid phenyl ester (CAPE) and zileuton.

Honey bee propolis is a good source of CAPE. Honey bee propolis exerts a number of beneficial effects.

These actions include:

- Anti-inflammatory action

---

[10] https://www.hindawi.com/journals/mi/2017/6904634/

- Antiviral
- Anticancer
- Antibacterial

The role of 5-lipoxygenase inhibitors in the treatment of lymphoedema.

5-lipoxygenase (5-LO) is a key enzyme in the synthesis of leukotrienes. Its importance as a therapeutic target cannot be underestimated.

5-LO brings about the first two steps of the transformation of arachidonic acid to leukotrienes.

However, the only clinically approved inhibitor of 5-lipoxygenase – zileuton – has unacceptable side effects.

There are some naturally occurring 5-lipoxygenase inhibitors. These include:

- Caffeic acid phenpropyl ester (found in bee propolis)
- Diphenlethyl ester*
- Phenylpropyl*
- Hypericum perforatum
- Gamma tocotrienol
- Delta tocopherol
- Gamma tocopherol
- Curcumin
- Erucic acid
- Monoenoic fatty acids
- Pumpkin seeds

We shall look at these – and others - in more detail later.

The starred substances above were found[11] to be significantly greater in inhibitory action than the reference molecules – which also showed 5-lipoxygenase inhibitory action. These comprised, caffeic acid phenyl ester (CAPE) and zileuton.

Honey bee propolis is a good source of CAPE. Honey bee propolis exerts a number of beneficial effects.

These include:

- Anti-inflammatory action
- Antiviral
- Anticancer
- Antibacterial

Monoenoic fatty acids

---

[11] https://www.hindawi.com/journals/mi/2017/6904634/

A number of long chain monoenoic fatty acids were found to have an effect on 5-LO activity. The results [12]show that oleic acid found in olive oil has by far the greatest inhibitory effect on 5-LO. Oleic acid is a monounsaturated fatty acid that is found in goodly amounts in olive oil and macadamia nuts.

Effect of Fatty Acid Inhibition Relative to Position of the Point of Unsaturation

| Fatty acid | Inhibition (%) | | | | Chain length | Number of carbons from double bond to: | |
| | 2.5 | 5.0 | 10 | 20 | | Terminal | Carboxyl |
	--------(μmoles)--------						
Oleic	48	66	77	89	18	9	9
Ricinoleic	17	35	67	90	18	9	9
Petroselinic	25	44	67	84	18	12	6
Vaccenic (*cis*)	40	70	83	92	18	7	11
5-*cis*-Eicosenoic	0	1	4	37	20	15	5
11-*cis*-Eicosenoic	25	40	62	81	20	9	11
Erucic	21	40	66	88	22	9	13
Nervonic	68	74	83	91	24	9	15

---

[12] https://link.springer.com/article/10.1007%2FBF02534605

It is no hardship using olive oil in salad dressings, pouring a tablespoon over meals or dipping a sandwich in a small amount before eating.

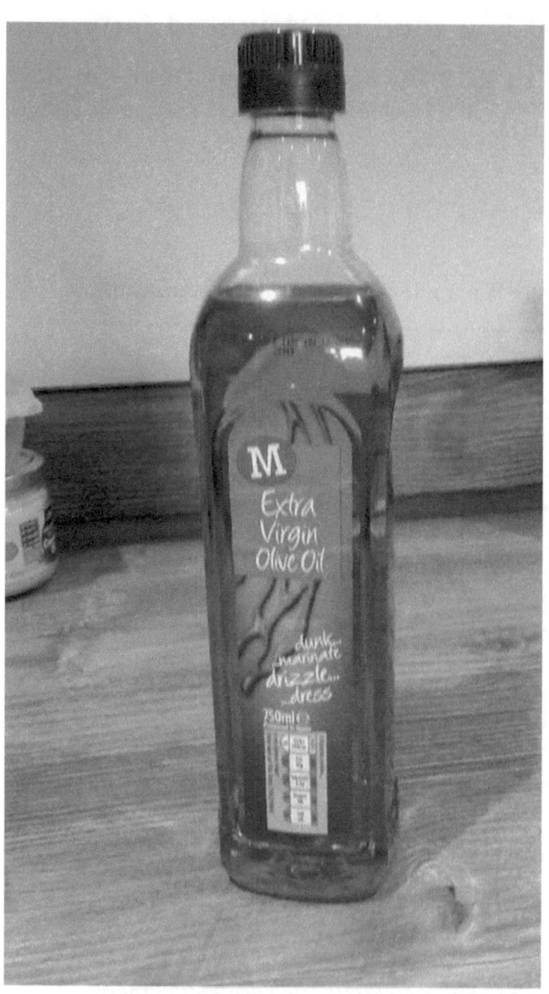

Erucic acid is mainly found in rapeseed oil. However, it is also found in many ornamental flowers such as nasturtiums and wallflowers.

In a study[13] erucic acid was found to competitively inhibit both peanut and soy bean lipoxygenases.

However, at high doses, erucic acid can damage the heart. Erucic acid may be eaten in small amounts though. Indeed, as it is added to many takeaway, ready meals and snacks, it is difficult to avoid and already forms a part of many people's diets, unwittingly or not. What we need to avoid is the excessive use of rapeseed oil. I would even go one step further and state that due to the inflammatory effects of the PUFA's they should be used with extreme caution, if at all. The liberal use of them, in just about any prepared food, has the potential for

[13]

https://onlinelibrary.wiley.com/doi/pdf/10.1007/BF02534605

by AJ St. Angelo - 1984

cancer, heart disease, arthritis and many other diseases as well as lymphoedema.

Many keen gardeners will know the ease with which nasturtiums can grow. In fact, the poorer the soil, the better. All parts of the nasturtium are edible including leaves, flowers and seeds. They look good tossed in salads and impart a peppery fresh flavour to the salad bowl. These are potentially a good source of erucic acid if you

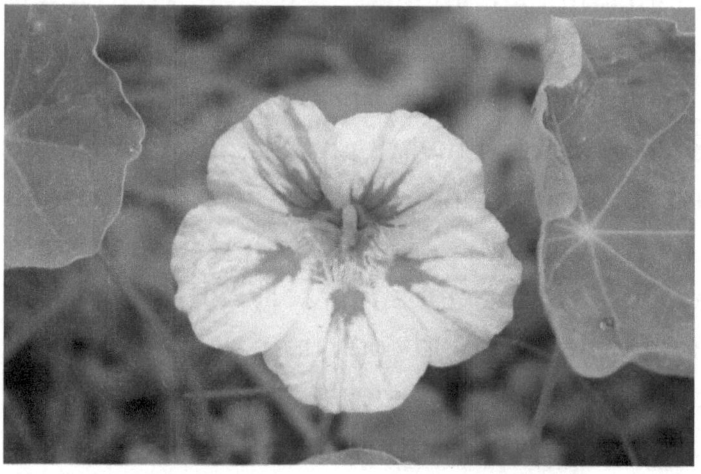

Nasturtiums come in a wide range of cheerful colours.

do not eat a diet that is already full of it and you wish to add a little as a 5-LO inhibitor.

<h2 style="text-align:center">Other 5-LO Inhibitors</h2>

Lycopene and saw palmetto

Studies[14] have also shown that lycopene and saw palmetto extract also help to suppress 5-LO.

Lycopene is the antioxidant that gives tomatoes their red colour. The Mediterranean diet contains fresh fruit and vegetables with plenty of olive oil. It is a diet which would benefit those who have lymphoedema.

Caffeic acid is another 5-LO inhibitor which is found in a wide range of foods. Its main source

---

[14] Agarwal S, Rao AV. Tomato lycopene and its role in human health and chronic diseases. CMAJ. 2000 Sep 19;163(6):739-44.

is coffee but its name 'caffeic' has absolutely nothing to do with caffeine.

Good sources of caffeic acid are:

- Wine
- Turmeric
- Coffee
- Herbs such as basil, oregano, sage, thyme
- Apples
- Cabbage
- Strawberries
- Mushrooms
- Cauliflower
- Kale
- Pears
- Olive oil

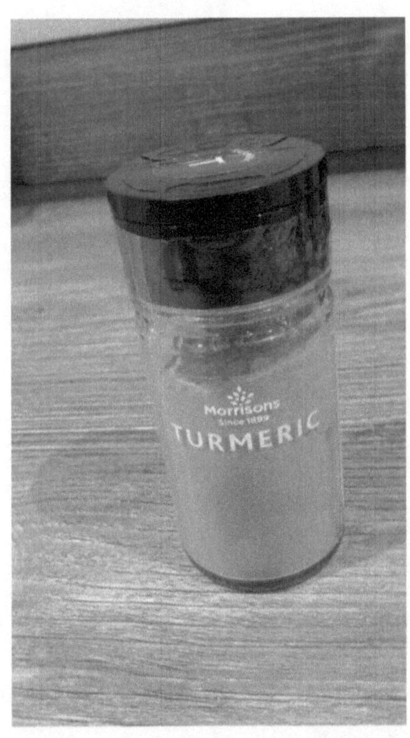

The active ingredient in turmeric, curcumin, is a 5-LO inhibitor.

Hypericum perforatum

A study[15] has found that naturally occurring analogues of hyperforin, that are isolated from H, perforatum, showed that oxidised hyperforin has efficacy against 5-LO.

---

[15] https://www.ncbi.nlm.nih.gov/pubmed/16787324

The study was conducted on intact human polymorphnuclear leukocytes – a type of white blood cells.

Vitamin E

Studies[16] have shown that the end products of vitamin E limit inflammation by targeting 5-LO.

Vitamin E is actually a mixture of eight naturally derived substances. They are fat soluble antioxidants that help to prevent the damage to cellular lipids that occurs in lymphoedema. However, they also have anti-inflammatory effects which are not attributed to their antioxidant properties.

A vitamin E deficiency can result in severe degenerative disease, atherosclerosis and a poor immune response. It was found that when alpha tocopherol was supplemented above the recommended daily allowance which is 400 IU's then there was a marked anti-inflammatory, anti-atherosclerotic and anti- tumour efficacy.

---

[16] https://www.nature.com/articles/s41467-018-06158-5

This study was carried out on animals.

There are three types of vitamin E whose metabolites show good efficacy against 5-LO. These are:

- Gamma tocopherol
- Delta tocopherol
- Gamma tocotrienol

Some of the metabolites of vitamin E are shown in the table overleaf.

Pumpkin seeds contain vitamin E and this may account for their inhibitory action on lipoxygenase.

Table[17] showing some of the inhibitory activity of vitamin E derivatives against 5-LO in cell-free and ...s.

	T				TE			
	α (a)	β (b)	γ (c)	δ (d)	α (e)	β (f)	γ (g)	δ (h)
Human recombinant 5-LO								
Vitamin E (1)	>1	0.75±0.15	0.91±0.15	0.31±0.10	0.33±0.08	0.19±0.03	0.20±0.06	0.17±0.1(
13'-CH$_2$OH (2)	0.35±0.04			0.12±0.04	0.11±0.01	0.09±0.03		0.15±0.0(
12'a-CH$_2$OH (3)							0.12±0.03	0.14±0.0(
13'-COOH (4)	0.27±0.01			>1	0.46±0.06	0.15±0.04	0.30±0.10	0.04±0.0(
Activated PMNL								
Vitamin E (1)	808±159	57±2	502±199	85±5	277±90	95±5	132±33	60±15
13'-CH$_2$OH (2)	0.19±0.05			0.54±0.02	0.27±0.10	0.38±0.09		1.26±0.3(
12'a-CH$_2$OH (3)							0.14±0.02	0.22±0.0(
13'-COOH (4)	0.08±0.00			2.01±0.59	1.70±0.52	0.31±0.11	0.49±0.03	0.26±0.0(

IC$_{50}$ values (μM) are given as mean ± s.e.m.; n = 3 independent experiments.

Sources of vitamin E

The best sources of vitamin E are:

- Seeds – sesame, sunflower. For example
- Nuts – almonds, hazelnuts, peanuts

---

[17] https://www.nature.com/articles/s41467-018-06158-5/tables/1

- Vegetable oils – wheat germ, corn, soybean, safflower, for example.
- Green leafy vegetables such as kale, spinach, chard and broccoli.

However, oils are oxidised easily and, in doing so will produce inflammation. Keep oils cool and in the dark and use only once.

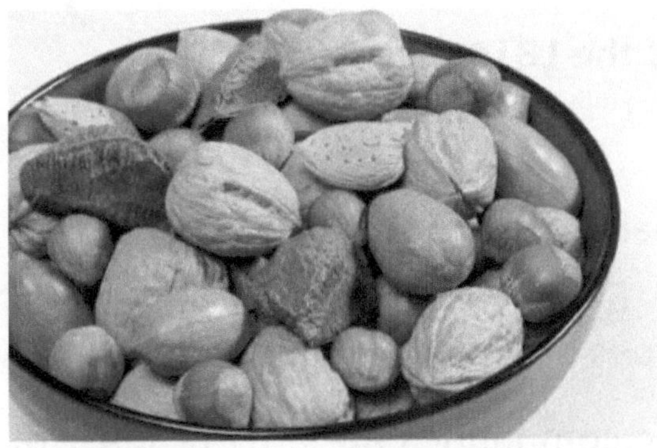

Nuts are an excellent source of vitamin E

Other targets of the LBT4 pathway to be considered in preventing the production of leukotrienes.

In order to reduce the possibility of leukotrienes being produced, we can also consider finding:

1. Antagonists of the LBT4 receptor (LBT4R) [18]
2. Inhibitors of the enzyme Leukotriene A4 Hydrolase (LA4H) as this enzyme helps generate LTB4.
3. Inhibitors of arachidonic acid release and leukotriene biosynthesis in human neutrophils

Antagonists of the LBT4 receptor

The main **antagonists of LBT4R** are tannins, gallic acid and calycosin. These are a types of phenolic compounds.

Phenolic compounds are a by-product of the amino acid, phenylalanine. They are a small molecule found in plants, including fruit and vegetables. Although

---

[18] Receptors are tiny shapes on a cell that attach to specific substances. In the case of LBT4R, this receptor attaches to the leukotriene B4 or its analogues.

they have known benefits for health they are not considered to be a nutrient.

Phenolic compounds can be divided into subgroups bases on slightly different chemical structure. The sub groups include:

- Tannins
- Flavonoids
- Coumarins
- Lignans

Depending on where these molecules are stored will further categorise them into soluble or bound forms.

Tannins are found in:

- Tea leaves
- Witch hazel
- Oak bark

Witch hazel is an astringent that is applied to the skin. It contains many compounds that are both powerful and effective. Witch hazel is antiviral and anti-inflammatory.

A study[19] found that using a lotion with 10% witch hazel extract was effective in reducing skin inflammation. It also reduced erythema (reddening of the skin that occurs alongside inflammation).

Gallic acid is not normally stable under food processing conditions. As such, its effectiveness, as an antioxidant may not be assured. However, it does have a number of food sources including:

- Cocoa
- Walnuts
- Hops
- Apples
- Flax seeds

Calycosin's main food sources are:

- Astragali (normally sold as a food supplement)

____

[19] https://www.ncbi.nlm.nih.gov/pubmed/11867970/

- Eggs
- Salmon

LTA4H inhibitor drugs - Ubenimex (Bestatin) - have not proven to reverse lymphoedema although it may have its uses in the early stages of lymphoedema.

Cannabinoid Oil

Cannabinoid is a potent analogue of LBT4 at a dose of 10mg/kg orally. Cannabinoid oil was found to inhibit LTB4 production in mouse blood. It has numerous other benefits.

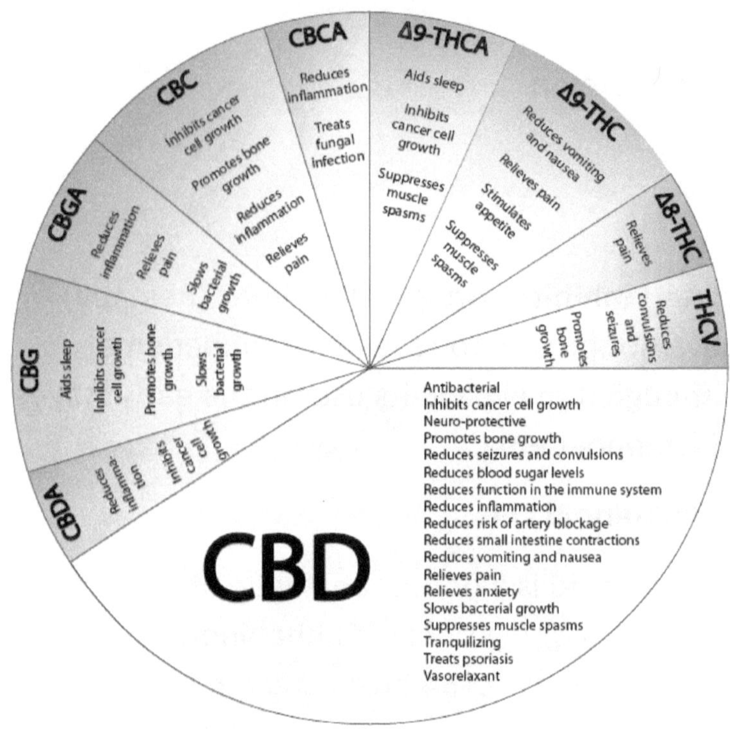

[20]

Natural suppressors of arachidonic acid and the D5D pathway

D5D is an enzyme. It causes production of either good or bad eicanosoids. If the D5D

---

[20] Cannabinoid oil Creative Commons Licence

enzyme is very active, then the production of arachidonic acid is higher resulting in the production of inflammatory eicanosoids. When insulin levels are raised this increases the activity of D5D. Simple carbohydrates increase insulin levels quite sharply. Simple carbohydrates are found in cakes, biscuits, white bread and other high sugar foods. This is one of the reasons why there is much marketing on the benefits of reducing them in the diet.

Fruit, while being marketed as being healthy due to its vitamin C content unfortunately contains fructose, a sugar which can raise blood sugar levels sharply.

Adenosine is a substance which is used to make adenosine triphosphate that helps transfer energy within cells. It is natural suppressor of arachidonic acid release and leukotriene biosynthesis. A potent natural source of adenosine is brewer's yeast. However, it competes with protein for absorption so it is better taken before food. As it also makes you feel sleepy – it is an inhibitory neurotransmitter – the perfect time to take it is before bedtime.

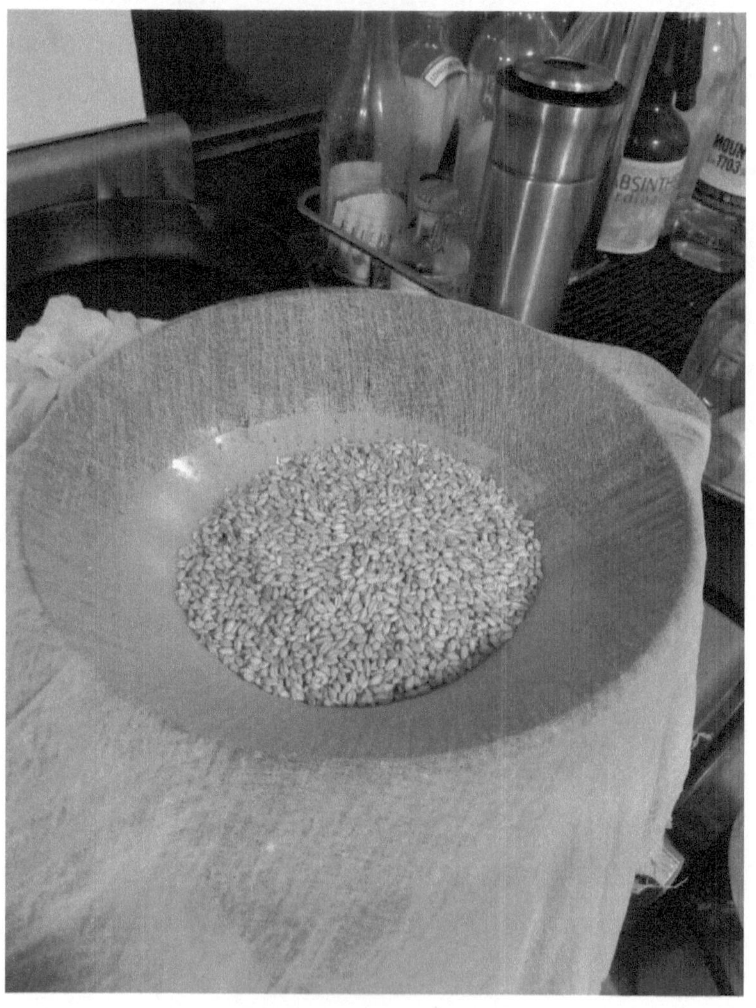

Brewers' yeast can be sprinkled over food. It is slightly bitter but a debittered type can be bought. It is also available in tablet form and is generally reasonable in price, however it comes. It is also a source of the vitamin B complex.

Other excellent sources of adenosine are:

- Liver and kidney (grass fed)
- Free range eggs
- Nuts and seeds
- Vegetables and fruit (however, due to the high fructose content of fruit, I recommend obtaining most of this from vegetables
- Omega three fatty acids –oily fish is the main source
- L-methionine found in onions and garlic
- Co-enzyme Q10 (main sources are offal but it is also found as a supplement in most good health food shops)

Eicosapentaenoic Acid

There is an omega 3 fatty acid called EPA (Eicosapentaenoic Acid) that inhibits the enzyme[21] [22] that produces arachidonic acid. The more EPA that you have in your diet the less arachidonic acid you will synthesise. In effect EPA reduces the amount of arachidonic acid and subsequently the pro-inflammatory prostaglandins, thromboxanes, eicosanoids and leukotrienes.

In a nutshell:

EPA reduces the synthesis of arachidonic acid by inhibiting the enzyme D5D

Reduced arachidonic acid = fewer inflammatory

- prostaglandins
- thromboxanes
- eicosanoids
- leukotrienes

---

[21] This enzyme is delta-5-desaturase (D5D)

[22] Sears B. The Zone. Regan Books. New York, NY (1995)

So to reduce leukotrienes we can now target two pathways:

1) The pathway that synthesises arachidonic acid by making sure that we have plenty of EPA in the diet and
2) The pathway that makes LTB4 leukotrienes from arachidonic acid by including 5-LO inhibitors in the diet.

DHA, another omega three fatty acid and closely associated with EPA does not have this effect. It is not an inhibitor of the D5D enzyme. It has a greater spatial size and cannot compete with arachidonic acid for the enzyme phospholipase A2 that helps release arachidonic acid from the cell membrane phospholipids where it is stored. Only EPA can do this.

 Interestingly, steroid therapy generally inhibits this D5D enzyme to reduce inflammation. However, EPA can do this but without the numerous side effects of steroids.

EPA also has an important part to play in reducing brain inflammation. However, it is rapidly oxidised so blood levels need to be kept high.

The main source of EPA is oily fish such as salmon, pilchards, mackerel and sardines. Oily fish needs to be eaten daily when lymphoedema is present. Failing this, supplementation is necessary as a preventative step in inhibiting the D5D enzyme that is necessary for the synthesis of arachidonic acid.

EPA, found in oily fish, is necessary in the battle against the synthesis of arachidonic acid and lymphoedema.

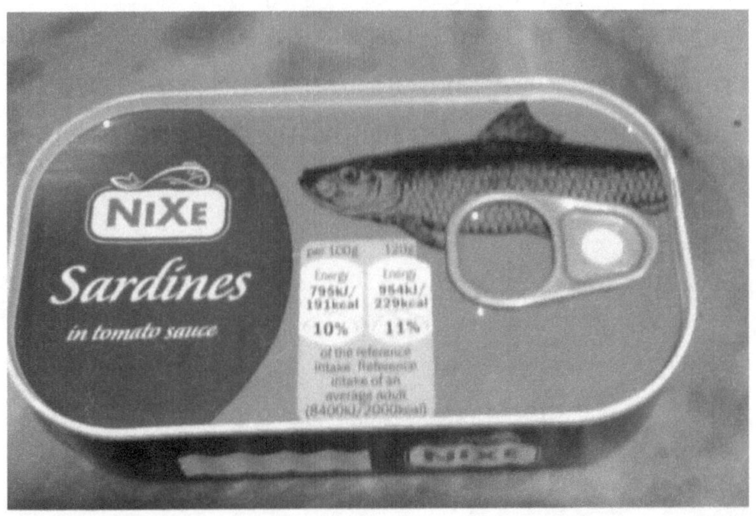

Cod liver oil is a great source of EPA, too.

Liquorice

When I refer to liquorice, I am not referring to that soft black stuff that you find in liquorice allsorts or formed into 'bootlaces' or 'straps' in red or black colours. No, the liquorice that I am referring to is the liquorice root of my childhood – something akin to fibrous twigs and only - I am assuming – slightly tastier.

These fibrous roots lasted a long time. You could chew or gnaw on them and there would still be enough for the following day and the day after that..............

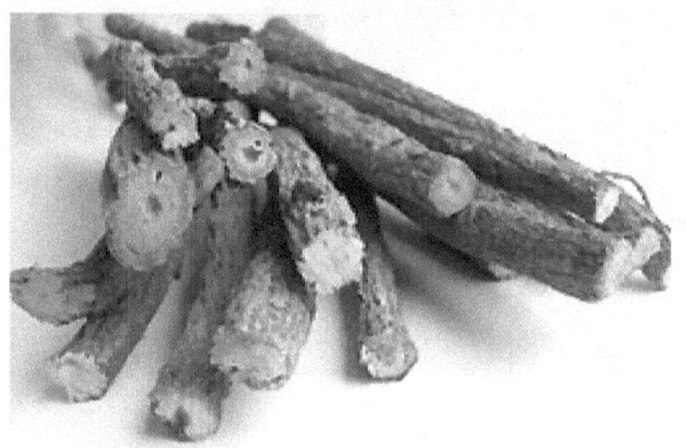

Mulethi Roots

Liquorice has 3 triterpenes, 13 flavonoids, exhibit anti-inflammatory properties mainly by decreasing TNF, NMP's PGE2 and free radicals. However, it does exhibit some effect on LTB4.

Triterpenes exhibit antidiabetic properties and therefore inhibit increases in insulin levels. Thus D5D is unlikely to be activated to such an extent that arachidonic acid is converted to inflammatory eicanosoids.

Boswellic acid

Boswellic acid is the active ingredient of frankincense. It has a number of anti-inflammatory properties. Studies[23] have shown tests using 11-keto-boswellic acid undertaken in vitro – that is outside a living organism - have demonstrated that it inhibits 5-lipoxygenase. However, when 800mg of frankincense extracts were given to human healthy volunteers, it failed to suppress leukotriene B4 plasma levels as it did in vitro test models. It is not clear why this is the case and studies on non-healthy people may be more enlightening.

---

[23] https://www.ncbi.nlm.nih.gov/pubmed/19374837

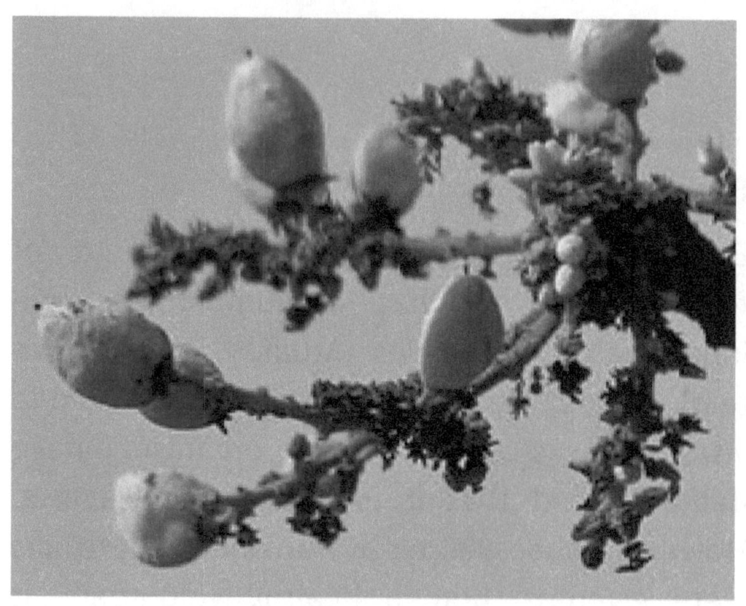

Boswellia comes from the resin of a plant Boswellia serrata

However, other studies have found that the premier natural 5-lo inhibitor is acetyl 11- keto – beta. That is, boswellia acid, also known as AKBA. It has superior ability to suppress the 5-LO enzyme and its leukotriene metabolites. It was found that the effect was increased if AKBA was taken with a little fat. This may be why the first study fell short.

In conclusion, boswellic acid may be useful for some people with lymphoedema. The interplay of genes may mean that boswellic acid is able to offer some benefit for some, if not all, patients with lymphoedema.

The effective dose has been found to be 50-60mg three times daily of up to 90% standard boswellia, daily. This good quality boswellia extract is vital in treating the lymphoedema. Most products available only contain 1-3% AKBA even though this is the active inflammatory ingredient.

The importance of leukotrienes and their impact on health cannot be underplayed. They are also implicated in a number of other disease states including:

- Asthma
- Allergies
- Colitis
- Arthritis
- Gastric disorder (ulcer formation

- Neurological disease (multiple sclerosis, Alzheimer's disease, motor neurone disease).

Leukotriene B4 is well known for damaging motor neurons.

LTB4 has been shown to promote insulin resistance in obese mice.

If you have any of the above medical conditions, then the risk of being diagnosed with others in the bulleted points does rise given that the underlying cause is the same. However, genes will also provide risk or protective factors. Therefore, any manifestations of this cluster of symptoms will differ among individuals due to genetic determination and every individual's own unique proximity to environmental triggers and protective factors.

Although it has been important to look at inhibitors of 5-LO, there are a number of activators of 5-LO which we ought to avoid if we want to prevent the initiation of inflammatory processes.

It is to this subject that I shall now turn.

Activators of 5-LO

Fatty acid hydroperoxides are potential activators of 5-LO. They are molecules that are derived primarily from fatty acids and steroids and are formed extensively by enzymes. However, it is possible to transform these intracellular hydro peroxides to hydroxides. This will limit the intensity and duration of the immune response involved in the chronic inflammation of lymphoedema.

How is this done? Well, Vitamin E is a radical scavenging agent. A study [24]has shown that vitamin E can donate a single electron to the process. When it does this the potentially harmful fatty acid hydro peroxides are converted to another substance – hydroxides - that do not activate 5-LO.

Glutathione peroxidases

---

[24] https://www.ncbi.nlm.nih.gov/pmc/articles/PMC5319403/

A class of enzymes known as glutathione peroxidases are responsible for reducing lipid peroxidases. The latter of which initiate inflammation.

Glutathione peroxidase is an intracellular enzyme. It can be found in the tissues of the body. The active site of this essential enzyme contains selenium.

Selenium is a trace element. It is found in variable amounts in food sources as the amount in food is determined by the amount of selenium in the soil that the food is grown in.

According to a review[25] over one billion people are suffering from a selenium deficiency.

Taking in enough selenium can also reduce the intensity and duration of the inflammation found in lymphoedema.

Good sources of selenium are:

---

[25] https://www.pnas.org/content/114/11/2848.full

- Yellow fin tuna
- Rice
- Beans
- Brazil nuts (two daily are all you need)
- Whole wheat bread

Of course, a little adaptation to the diet may be necessary in order to begin to reverse the chronic inflammation in lymphoedema but a diet for lymphoedema is not a difficult one to follow. There are few rules;

- take out the PUFA vegetable oils, wherever possible and use the saturated fats in their place.
- Use olive oil as it is a monounsaturated oil. However, you must not heat olive oil. Use it on salads liberally, dip your bread into it and, once used, store it in a cool, dark place.
- Add other 5-LO inhibitors into your diet as you are able and do try and avoid ready snacks and meals since it is hard to find any that do not include a PUFA.

- Make sure that you eat oily fish on a regular basis and/or supplement with EPA.
- Consider whether you are taking in optimum levels of minerals and vitamins so that the desaturase enzymes can respond accurately to the synthesis of pro or anti-inflammatory compounds.

Cellulitis

It would be remiss of me not to include a section on cellulitis and how we can keep this at bay while the lymphatic system is healing. Most people with lymphoedema will have already become acquainted with this debilitating infection. Cellulitis is a serious complication of lymphoedema. It can cause further damage to the lymphatic system setting up a cycle of increasing damage and infection.

Cellulitis is a serious infection of the skin and soft tissues. It is generally caused by the streptococcus or staphylococcus bacterium which enters the skin through a crack or break in the skin. This is why patients with lymphoedema are requested to moisturise their skin on a daily basis.

The incidence of methicillin resistant staphylococcus aureus (MRSA) is increasing.

Cellulitis occurs as the lymphatic system fails to function properly. This result in lymph collecting in the soft tissues of parts of the body such as the legs or arms. This collection of lymph is a rich breeding ground for pathogens.

Signs and symptoms of cellulitis include:

- Red, swollen, painful areas
- Warmth in the painful area
- Fever with or without chills

If the inflammation and swelling spreads rapidly then water blisters can appear – these blisters leak lymph from the skin.

Natural antimicrobials as a *preventative* or *adjunctive treatment* to antibiotics.

Zinc has a beneficial role to play in many other disease states. Studies have shown it to be effective in metabolic and chronic diseases that include: metabolic and chronic diseases such as diabetes, cancer, oesophageal cancer, breast cancer and neurodegenerative diseases.

Further evidence[26] exists for a link between zinc deficiency and a number of infectious diseases such as malaria, HIV, measles, pneumonia and tuberculosis.

---

[26] https://www.ncbi.nlm.nih.gov/pmc/articles/PMC5490603/

Zinc also has an important part to play in the health of skin and its underlying tissue. A study[27] found that zinc was important to:

- The integrity of the skin and wound repair
- It maintains macrophage and neutrophil functions (white blood cells which fight infection)
- Zinc maintains and activates Natural Killer activity and complement.

Complement proteins are part of the innate immune system – that which you had from birth. They enhance – or complement - the ability of antibodies and phagocytic cells to clear infective agents and damaged cells.

Complement proteins –of which there are nearly 60 – can be found in blood plasma or on the surfaces of cells.

Natural Killer cells are part of the innate immune system. That is, the immune system that you were born with. It migrates to

---

[27] https://www.hindawi.com/journals/drp/2014/709152/

infection sites and ingests any harmful substances like bacteria, cancerous cell and foreign particles.

They do this by attacking the infected cell membrane until it bursts and the contents leak out. The cell isn't viable at that point.

Natural killer cells are general in action and will attack anything that isn't part of self.

Zinc and inflammation are so tied up with lymphoedema that we ought to take a closer look at these.

Inflammation

There are some great old-fashioned remedies for inflammation.   Because some of the treatments can be found in the store cupboard many people do not believe that they have the effectiveness that they have.

In days gone by   people will have noticed that some common substances worked for pain or inflammation even though the underlying mechanism for the effect may not have been known at the time.

Some of these substances were just as good or even better than some drugs produced by big pharma's but they went out of fashion when treatments became the domain of the pharmaceutical industries and doctors. We have become used to believing that the only medications and treatments that will work are the ones that are prescribed for us.

One of these treatments will be found in every cupboard of those who bake from time to time. This amazing substance is bicarbonate of soda – also known as   sodium bicarbonate - is cheap and effective as an anti-inflammatory   agent.

Moreover, there is very good research to bear this out.

Researchers at the Medical College of Georgia discovered a nerve centre in a cell layer in the spleen that controls the immune response, and therefore inflammation, throughout the body. It is quelled by taking 2g of baking soda in water for two weeks. Can something be that simple? Well, yes it can.

When sodium bicarbonate is taken there is a shift from inflammatory to an anti-inflammatory profile which is systemic. It is quite probable that this shift is due to the pro-inflammatory cells being changed to anti-inflammatory ones. Additionally, there appears to be a greater production of anti-inflammatory macrophages. It was also found that there was an increased production of T cells which drive down the immune response and prevent autoimmunity.

The only downside to this taking sodium bicarbonate is that this has the potential to raise your blood pressure. If you do have raised blood pressure, then taking 250mg of magnesium and a glass of tomato juice for the potassium will most likely address this. In addition, both magnesium and potassium are anti-inflammatory in nature and so will enhance the actions of sodium bicarbonate on the cell layer in the spleen.

The Trace Element, Zinc

Zinc is a trace element which is often associated with the health of the immune system. Indeed, a zinc deficiency can lead to a vulnerability to infection. Zinc is better known for its ability to activate T lymphocytes. It also has a regulatory role in controlling the immune response as well as attacking cancerous and infected cell. Zinc supplementation studies in the elderly have shown a reduction in the rate and severity of infections, decreased oxidative stress and the presence of fewer inflammatory cytokines. However, its super status is not just confined to the health of the immune system. Nevertheless, when considering the inflammatory processes and infections that have been found to fuel lymphoedema, zinc's impact on health cannot be ignored.

Zinc is required for many functions in the body especially in relation to activating enzymes which speed up metabolic processes in the body. Some of these processes may be related to wound healing and age-related chronic diseases such as age-related macular degeneration. However, there are some quite remarkable effects on weight loss when a zinc deficiency is corrected. Obesity may contribute to the progression of lymphoedema since obesity is very much associated with inflammation. Since zinc deficiency is rife in society it is worth looking at the impact of zinc on weight and the underlying reasons why it might aid weight loss.

Zinc is essential for the smooth running of the thyroid gland. It is needed to produce thyroid stimulating hormone. The latter, if in short supply, results in low levels of the hormones T4 and T3. These hormones help regulate the body's metabolism turning food into energy. Without   the proper synthesis of these hormones not only will weight gain occur but the person who lacks these thyroid hormones will feel cold and tired.

Zinc supplements help to increase the weight loss on those on a calorie restricted diets. In a study, calorie reduction of 300Kj was undertaken by individuals supplemented with 30mg of zinc. The control group did not receive any supplementary zinc. This regime was followed for 15 weeks. After 15 weeks there was a significant reduction of body weight, BMI, waist circumference in the zinc supplemented group. In addition, it was found that there were lower levels of C-reactive protein, insulin resistance and appetite score.

Therefore, zinc appears to tackle obesity from different angles. Firstly, it helps correct any deficiency which might impact the metabolic rate. Secondly, it tackles insulin resistance enabling food to be used as an energy source instead of being used for fat storage. Thirdly, it aids appetite reduction and fourthly it helps tackle inflammation.

Many comorbid conditions occur alongside obesity. Oxidative stress underlies the molecular mechanisms responsible for the development of many inflammatory diseases like atherosclerosis, diabetes mellitus, rheumatoid arthritis as well as neurodegenerative disorders. The cellular antioxidant system proves insufficient to remove the reactive oxygen species which damage cells and create inflammation in this process. It would not be unusual to find many other inflammatory conditions comorbid with lymphoedema.

The regulatory function of zinc cannot be underestimated. It is essential to the structure and function of nearly 3000 macromolecules and over 300 enzymes.

Macromolecules are very large molecules such as proteins made from amino acids.

Common macromolecules, monomers and some end products are:

MACROMOLECULE	MONOMERS (the building blocks)	END PRODUCT
protein	Amino acids	Protein – many types such as keratin for hair and collagen for connective tissue, enzymes and antibodies.
Nucleic acids	Nucleotides	RNA and DNA
Lipids	Fatty acids	Fats, sterols, waxes and oils

Although Zinc is known for its antiviral impact, it also has a beneficial effect on secretory molecules and the bactericidal activity of human peptidoglycan recognition proteins. (PGLYRP's)

Peptidoglycan is a substance that forms the cell walls of bacteria. Streptococcus and staphylococcus bacteria are responsible for the soft tissue infection, cellulitis. The ability of the immune system to detect bacteria – and thus deal with it – is partially dependent on the available serum zinc.

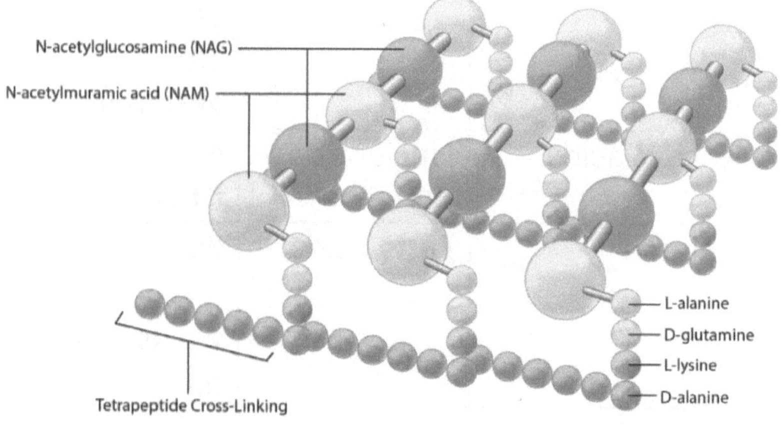

Structure of peptidoglycan. Note the amino acids required for its synthesis

The importance of having adequate daily amounts of zinc cannot be underestimated. Zinc has been described as the element with a minor plasma pool and a rapid turnover.

There are certain groups of individuals that are more susceptible to zinc deficiency. These include:

- Diabetics
- Cancer patients
- Those with liver disease
- Those on a high plant diet as the phytates in plants bind to zinc
- Those on high copper or high iron diets
- Those who are on a calorie reducing diet
- Those who are under stress
- The elderly
- Breast fed babies
- Pregnant women
- Alcoholism
- Those with malabsorption problems of the digestive tract such as Crohn's disease.
- Anyone who is susceptible to soft tissue injury and infection.

Sources of zinc include:

- Oysters (very high in zinc) 3 ounces provides 673% of the daily value
- Beef – 3 ounces provide 65% of your daily requirements
- Beef patty – 3 ounces provides 64% of your daily requirement
- Baked beans – half a cup provides 26% of your daily requirement.

The benefits of zinc for lymphoedema and its related comorbidities cannot be understated.

The Daily Requirement of Zinc has been placed at:

Men – 11g

Women 8mg

However, for short periods of no greater than a month, upwards of this amount may be used to aid the processes which counteract lymphoedema. Any longer and you raise the risk of iron and copper depletion which carry their own risk of deficiency diseases. In matters of cellulitis then should it occur then 100mg of zinc can be taken immediately followed by 25mg of zinc until the infection is controlled.

Given the seriousness of the infection cellulitis, then recourse to antibiotics should never be discounted. However, antibiotics do have serious side effects and may impair the immune system by their negative impact on the gut microbiota.

Alterations to gut microbial communities are able to cause immune dysregulation and autoimmune disorders. Optimum gut microbial communities stimulate the development of innate and acquired component. In addition, gut microbiota synthesises vitamins B1, B2, B5, B6, folic acid, biotin and vitamin k.

Making sure that your diet is zinc adequate from the outset may make sure that you never have cellulitis.

Personal anecdote of the effect of zinc on the immune system

My husband who is normally healthy, started suffering with sneezing, lethargy and cold symptoms. However, he maintained he was 'fine' so I didn't offer him any alternative medicine. By day four he felt, and looked, very poorly. His chest was rattling.

I, at this stage, started coming down with the same symptoms. I wasn't too happy about this so I took 50mg of zinc and gave my husband the same amount. My symptoms subsided overnight so that, by the morning I was back to normal and my husband was much improved.

Zinc is one of those trace elements that should be kept in the medicine kit for times such as these. People who abstain from eating red meats as well as vegetarians and vegans are at a high risk of developing zinc deficiency as the amounts of zinc in plant based foods is insufficient to maintain adequate levels in the body. Further, a diet that contains mainly non-digestible plant ligands such as phytates, some dietary fibres

Phytates are antioxidant compounds found in whole grains, legumes, nuts and seeds. They can bind to zinc (as well as other dietary minerals) and slow or inhibit their absorption

and lignin inhibit the absorption of zinc.

According to WHO[28], zinc deficiency is currently the fifth leading cause of mortality and morbidity in developing countries. It is estimated that it affects about one-third of the world's population.

---

[28] World Health Organisation. The World Health Report. World Health Organization; Geneva, Switzerland: 2002.

Staphylococcus aureus[29]

Approximately 25% of the population are long term carriers of staphylococcus aureus (*S. aureus*). It is found in normal skin flora, in the lower reproductive tract of women and in the nostrils.

S aureus can produce a wide range of medical conditions including boils, cellulitis, pimples, abscesses, folliculitis and carbuncles, among others. However, it can also produce more severe infections which can be life threatening. These include:

- Meningitis
- Osteomyelitis
- Endocarditis
- Sepsis
- Toxic shock syndrome

---

[29] Treat Infection Naturally by Lynne D M Noble

S. aureus is one of the most common causes of hospital acquired infections and is generally the cause of wound infections following surgery. Thousands of deaths each year are *S. aureus* related with the elderly and those with compromise immune systems being mostly at risk.

S. aureus employs a number of defensive weapons which it uses to become resistant to many antibiotics. For example, staphylococcal resistance to penicillin is mediated by an enzyme, penicillinase. This cleaves part of the ring of the penicillin molecule which renders it effective. There are *B* lactam antibiotics such as flucloxacillan which are able to resist degradation by staphylococcal penicillinase.

Fortunately, coconut oil is effective against *S. aureus*.

The recommended dosage of coconut oil during illness is 4-8 tablespoonsful daily. This can be stirred into fruit juice to make It more palatable if this is preferred.

Vitamin B3 (Nicotinamide)

Studies have shown that vitamin B3 may be able to combat some of the antibiotic resistant staphylococcal infections.

Research has shown that high doses of this vitamin increased by up to 1,000 times the ability of the immune cells to kill staphylococcal bacteria.

These findings were published in the *Journal of Clinical Investigation* on August 27 by researchers from the Linus Pauling Institute at Oregon State University, UCLA and other institutions.

Vitamin B3 stimulates the innate immune system to provide a much more powerful response. In the case of vitamin B3, clinical doses of this increased the numbers and effectiveness of neutrophils. These white blood cells kill and eat harmful bacteria.

NEUTROPHIL

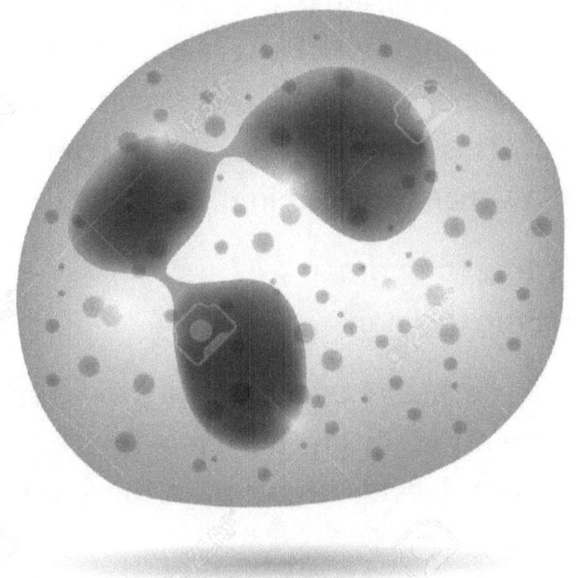

Further studies showed that clinical doses of vitamin B3 appeared to wipe out the staph infection in only a few hours.

It is not recommended that megadoses of this vitamin are taken routinely, without medical supervision, since high doses of vitamin B3 can damage the liver.

Given the potential negative side effects of mega doses of vitamin B3, a healthy balanced diet containing whole grains, mushrooms, peanuts, avocados and green peas should be the aim. This will provide the recommended daily allowance for vitamin B3 of

- 14mg for women
- 16mg for men.

Higher doses are available via prescription but are normally given to help lower cholesterol levels rather than to treat staph infections.

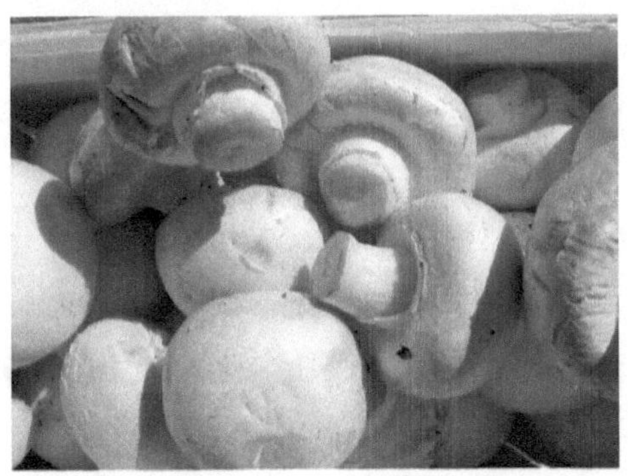

Mushrooms contain vitamin B3 and can help fight staphylococcus infections.

Riboflavin (vitamin B2)

Studies[30] into the effectiveness of riboflavin found that, along with antibiotics, it helps to balance reactive oxygen species and inflammatory cytokines. Riboflavin also controls *Staphylococcus aureus* (one of the cellulitis causing bacterium). Riboflavin was found to boost (murine) macrophage function and regulate inflammation.

---

[30] https://www.ncbi.nlm.nih.gov/pubmed/27932936

Oleuropeins

Studies have shown that oleuropeins at a low concentration of 1% delayed growth of *S. aureus* and that higher concentrations (0.4-0.6%) inhibited growth completely.

Oleuropeins are found in olives and olive oil and as well as inhibiting the growth of *s. aureus* has already established itself as a lipoxygenase inhibitor. Oleuropeins not only protects against bacteria by dissolving the lining of micro-organisms but also protects against insects. This is a further reason to include olive oil daily in the diet!

Streptococcus pyogenes

A number of studies[31] have shown that phenolic compounds - like thymol and

---

[31]

https://www.microbiologyresearch.org/docserver/fulltext/jmm/56/4/519.pdf?expires=1552400098&id=id&accname=guest&checksum=CC420816FFB634E6E4D13F5FA15A44C8

carvacrol - found in herbs such as oregano and thyme have significant bactericidal activity. These phenolic compounds have the ability to interact with the bi-lipid layer of the bacterial cell membranes and punch holes in them. This causes loss of cell membrane integrity and allows leakage of cellular material thus disrupting the bacterium's ability to flourish.

Lactoferrin

Strangely, lactoferrin is found in tears, human milk – more than bovine milk products- saliva and nasal secretions. As an important multi-functional protein it is found on all mucosal surfaces where it kills staphylococcus aureus. However, lactoferrin is found in the fat globules of milk products so those individuals who use only skimmed milk or low fat milk products will not benefit from this natural antibiotic.

Mushrooms

Mushrooms are thought to be one of the richest sources of natural antibiotics. It is thought that they evolved this way as they had to protect themselves from the often damp and dirty environment that they grow in.

Many prescribed antibiotics are made from mushrooms. These include streptomycin and tetracycline. For example, Ganomycin, a powerful antibiotic is made from Reishi mushrooms. However, most mushrooms will have both antibacterial and antiviral properties although these will be of greater or lesser strength depending on the variety of mushroom.

While not every individual likes mushrooms where they are not objected to, then their immune boosting properties should be harnessed as often as possible especially where the possibility of recurrent infection is high.

 Irradiated mushrooms also contain excellent amounts of vitamin D. Vitamin D is required for the synthesis of an antimicrobial known as cathelicidin so irradiated mushrooms also help fight infection through another channel.

Mushrooms also contain excellent amounts of selenium- a trace mineral that is required in the synthesis of glutathione peroxidases that helps reduce inflammatory responses. Mushrooms are an excellent food source for individuals with lymphoedema. Their versatility is second to none and they can be added to:

- Mushroom loaf
- Soups
- Sauces
- Stuffings

Their versatility is limited only by the imagination.

The Role of Fasting in Reducing Chronic Inflammation

A recent article that appeared in the Medical Express has highlighted the importance of fasting in reducing inflammation and chronic inflammatory disease.

As we have already discovered lymphoedema is a chronic inflammatory disease which has the potential to respond to such measures. Even more exciting is the discovery that fasting does not affect the immune systems response to acute infections.

Calorie restriction has long been known to improve inflammatory and auto immune disease but how this comes about has only been discovered.

Apparently, intermittent fasting reduces the release of monocytes. These are pro-inflammatory cells which are found circulating in the blood. During fasting these cells go into a dormant state and become less inflammatory in the process.

Monocytes are highly inflammatory and can cause serious tissue damage. Dr Merad[32] explained that increasing amounts of monocytes can be seen in the blood circulation of populations over the last few centuries due to different eating patterns.

Further studies have shown that people who have a poor diet can ameliorate the effects by the periodic use of a low calorie, plant based diet. This causes the cells to act like the body is fasting.

____

[32] https://medicalxpress.com/news/2019-08-fasting-inflammation-chronic-inflammatory-diseases.html

Longo[33] and colleagues conducted clinical trials where participants were allowed to consume between 750and 1l00 calories daily over a five day period. The diet contained specific proportions of proteins, fats and carbohydrates. The participants saw reduced risk factors for many life threatening diseases.

'Fasting is hard to stick to and it can be dangerous. We know that the fasting-mimicking diet is safer and easier than water only fasting, but the big surprise from this study is that if you replace the fasting-mimicking diet, which includes pre-biotic ingredients, with water, we don't see the same benefits.

In mice studies, these findings were replicated. In the study one group of mice adhered to a four-day fasting-mimicking diet by consuming approximately 50 percent of their normal caloric intake on the first day and 10 per cent of their normal caloric intake from the second through fourth days. Another group fasted with

---

[33]

https://www.sciencedaily.com/releases/2019/03/190306171247.htm

a water based diet only for 48 hours. The fasting-mimicking diet was found to mitigate or reverse some of the inflammatory processes while the water based fast did not. This indicated that certain nutrients in the fasting-mimicking diet contributed to the positive changes found in the plant based fast.

The conclusion formed was that 'fasting primes the body for improvement, but it is the re-feeding that provides the opportunity to rebuild cells and tissues.'

The vital nutrient in the battle for weight reduction

Weight reduction is part of the fight in reducing the impact of lymphoedema. It is also a hard fight since when we reduce calories and body mass decreases, the synthesis of the hunger inhibiting hormone, leptin, is also reduced. As a result, hunger pangs increase and it is not long before the diet is abandoned without achieving its aims.

How then can we lose weight without damaging muscle mass and further, making sure that this is undertaken without too much effort on our part. Food is meant to be enjoyed and there is little enjoyment in it when every calorie is being counted on a day to day basis.

Well, the answer is that the fasting is undertaken only intermittently, and for short periods, and is therefore not damaging in the way that longer and often ill thought calorie restriction can be.

 In addition, a recently discovered nutritional substance which is present in some foods has been found to be the dieter's best friend. Its name is choline and some choline is made in the body but most has to be provided in the food that we eat. Unfortunately, most people are deficient in this vitamin like substance.

What does choline do to help weight loss? Well, choline has been found to help the body use fat as a fuel and further, choline helps to remove excess fat from the blood. When fat is used as a fuel then hunger will not occur.

Studies[34] on the effect of choline supplementation on rapid weight loss and biochemical variables among female taekwondo and judo athletes have born this out. For a number of reasons, it is necessary for athletes to lose weight before important matches. This is undertaken using a number of nutritional

---

[34] https://www.ncbi.nlm.nih.gov/pmc/articles/PMC4096089/#b4-jhk-40-77

substances of which one is choline. Dramatic weight loss without the loss of muscle mass has been observed in those taking choline supplementation.

The athletes took 2g of choline daily divided into two 1g doses for one week. The results indicated a 10.23% change in loss of body fat. The results support the hypothesis that choline could be used to lose weight rapidly without detriment to other body systems.

Good sources of choline are eggs and liver. Two eggs provide about half of the choline requirements for the day.

A Recommended Daily Allowance has not been established for choline since it is a fairly newly discovered substance. However, an Adequate Intake has been established and this is:

- 425mg for women
- 550mg for men

Some individuals will require less than this and others more. There are a number of groups of people who are likely to require more and, as such be at risk of being deficient in choline. These groups are:

- Anyone with a poor diet or malabsorption problems
- Pregnant mothers
- Nursing mothers
- The elderly
- Vegetarians and vegans

The best sources of choline are foods which are now advised as those that may increase cholesterol levels. As such they are avoided. In addition, the best source of choline – beef liver - has fallen out of popularity. When we take eggs and liver out of the diet then it can be seen that achieving the adequate intake of choline is not easy.

Foods containing choline

- One large egg: 120mg
- Beef liver: one slice contains 280mg
- Salmon: 4 ounces contains 65mg
- Cod: 85gms contains 250mg
- Cauliflower: 120ml contains 25mg

- Broccoli: 120ml contains 24mg
- Brussels sprouts: one cup cooked 65mg
- Soybean oil: one tablespoon contains 47mg
- Peanut butter: one tablespoon 10mg

It can be see that it is considerably harder to obtain adequate intakes of choline in a plant based diet than it is for those who include meat in their meals.

There is no fear in eating eggs. One of Choline's functions is to lower cholesterol levels and as eggs contain superb amounts of choline then the hype that they can contribute to heart disease and stroke is unfounded. Choline can also lower blood pressure.

It makes sense to increase levels of choline in the diet. This is not an overly difficult thing to achieve. For example, stirring a couple of egg yolks into mashed potato before topping a shepherd's pie or making proper Crème Anglaise with egg yolks goes well towards the Adequate Intake of choline. Making a shepherd's pie with minced liver is also a tried and tested recipe in our household. I make this with lamb's liver as the flavour is more delicate than that of beef liver. However, it depends on individual taste. Liver is such a good all round food that it is eaten twice weekly in our house.

If cooking is not your forte, then supplements are useful and easily obtainable online and in health food stores. It is recommended   that no more than 600mg is taken daily but be guided by the instructions on the pack.

Putting it all together

It is clear that nutrition plays a huge part in the instigation and progression of disease states. Diets have changed a great deal. We are beleaguered by fast food and ready meals; these are sources of PUFA's omega 6's which contain arachidonic acid. Snacking on energy bars and crisps, eating 'healthy' granola have become a way of life. Most of our poultry, beef and eggs are not grass fed any more. They are commercially raised on corn products. This increases the intake of arachidonic acid with the potential for its metabolites to form pro-inflammatory leukotriene that potentiates lymphoedema. The pro inflammatory effects of commercially raised meat is one of the reasons that the produce of grass fed cattle and poultry is seen as superior. We do need arachidonic acid but not in the quantities that we are now being unwittingly force fed - and with all the consequences that has for our health.

Surgery and cancer therapy might increase the risk for lymphoedema but if the enzymes that help synthesise arachidonic acid or transform it to LTB4 is inhibited, then the inflammation and subsequent damage to the lymphatic system that takes place in lymphoedema cannot occur. Indeed, raised levels of omega 6 PUFA's and, desaturase enzymes are also risk factors for breast cancer.

Until pharmacological companies are able to produce a safe 5-LO inhibitor then the patient must consider:

- Reducing the amount of arachidonic acid in their diet with a serious emphasis on decreasing the amount of the omega 6 poly unsaturated fatty acid oils eaten.
- In addition, regular amounts of EPA – an omega 3 fatty acid – should be included in the diet.

- Regularly including 5-LO inhibitors in the diet as well as considering supplementation.
- Reducing the amount of 5-LO activators
- Increasing the amount of minerals and vitamins that are required to enable the desaturase enzymes to respond appropriately to prevailing conditions

To give you an idea of how this might play out in meals, I have included a couple of recipes at the end of this book that include 5-LO inhibitors. Recipes for oily fish are not included since most people, if they eat fish, will have their favourite recipes anyway.

EPA supplements – often accompanied by DHA – are easily found in health food stores and supermarkets as is cod liver oil. While DHA is unlikely to Impact the chronic inflammation found in lymphoedema, in the way that EPA does, it is unlikely to be found in isolation from EPA. Nevertheless, DHA has many health benefits so supplements that contain both DHA and EPA can be used if you don't want to source a single supplement of EPA.

 The Dangers of Manufactured Citric Acid (MCA)

As always, there can be more than one cause of any manifestation of a condition. During my research I happened to have my attention drawn to Manufactured Citric Acid and spent weeks following this through as it seemed to have implications for many chronic diseases such asthma, lymphoedema, lipoedema, Alzheimer's disease, arthritis, allergies and gastrointestinal disturbance. This is not a definitive list. Indeed, my attention was first turned towards the problems with MCA when I was advising someone on the benefits of real – not manufactured citric acid – in aiding gut motility.

The discovery of citric acid was credited to an alchemist Jabir ibn Hayaan going as far back at the 8th century. However, it was not isolated in

99

its pure form until nine centuries later when Carl Steele crystallised it from lemon juice in 1784.

The lemon juice was imported from Italy and peak production occurred in 1915-1916 after which it began to decline due to cost.

The change from the crystallisation of citric to a fermentation process occurred in 1919 in Belgium using the mould known as penicillium. However, the duration of fermentation and the risk of contamination meant that the use of penicillium was abandoned.

In 1917, James Currie — an American food chemist — discovered that the mould *Aspergillus niiger* could produce cost effective amounts of citric acid using molasses as the raw material.

In 1919, Pfizer adopted this method and began to produce citric acid using *Aspergillus niger*. This method is used today and we refer to this citric acid as manufactured citric acid or MCA.

The Food Standards Agency normally evaluates food additives for safety and they are given

GRAS status – Generally Recognised as Safe. However, the Food Additives Amendment 1958 excluded any additives – including MCA – that were in use before 1958 that had not appeared to have demonstrated harm.

This does not mean that it does not cause harm. Some conditions take many years to diagnose and even so, the underlying cause may still be unknown.

99% of citric acid used today is the MCA sort. It is an ubiquitous substance and arguably the most common food additive. It is used to stabilise and preserve the active ingredients.

The global market growth and the related use of citric acid is undoubtedly driven by concomitant growth in pharmaceuticals, cosmetics and processed foods.

It can be found in:

Processed and prepared foods

Carbonated beverages, fruit and energy drinks

Nutritional supplements and vitamins

Common snacks

Confectionary

Pharmaceuticals

Canned fruit and veg

It is also used in non-food stuffs as it is a useful disinfectant against many viruses and bacteria.

Currently, the market share of MCA appears to be taken by:

Food and beverages	70%
Pharmaceuticals and cosmetics	20%
Cleaning and softening agents	10%

In a research paper[35] the potential harms of MCA are raised. The authors cite four case reports of individuals who demonstrate symptoms which include:

---

[35] https://www.ncbi.nlm.nih.gov/pmc/articles/PMC6097542/

Joint pain with swelling and stiffness, muscular pain, dyspnea, abdominal cramping, and enervation that started within 2-12 hours of ingesting anything which contained MCA.

The severity of symptoms appears to be the deciding factor in how long before they resolve which could be anywhere from 8-72 hours.

The case participants did not know beforehand which foods contained MCA yet were able to correctly identify, based on symptoms, those which were.

It was found that the ingestion of natural forms of citric acid did not result in such symptoms.

Aspergillus niger is thermos tolerant and cannot be killed. Even when it is the end products is still pro-inflammatory. It is extremely likely that there are contaminants from production.

China is the largest producer of MCA and continues to expand as demand expects. Auto immune disorders and allergies have been found to be increasing in parallel.

Indeed, some of other conditions that appear to be related to MCA ingestion are:

ASD, juvenile idiopathic arthritis, fibromyalgia, lymphoedema as well as allergies and angieoedema type conditions and neurological conditions.

Late onset Alzheimer's disease is associated with reduced nicotinamide adenosine triphosphate (NAD) metabolism and an altered citric acid cycle also known as the TCA or the tricarboxylic acid cycle.

As it is MCA that is found in pharmaceutical drugs, then the impact of taking such drugs cannot be ignored.

Serious side effects are outlined[36] and include the citric acid which forms part of potassium citrate and sodium citrate too. This include numbness, tingly feeling, swelling or rapid weight gain, muscle twitching, cramps, fast or slow heartbeat, confusion, mood changes, bloody or tarry stools, severe stomach pain, ongoing diarrhoea or seizures.

---

[36] https://www.uofmhealth.org/health-library/d03951a1

Given MCA's potential for inflammation - in susceptible people - which would impede the movement of lymph and its ubiquitous nature then removing MCA from the diet entirely for one week would be a wise move in order to ascertain if MCA is contributing to your condition.

Recipes

This book is not meant to be a complete recipe book in itself. The 'diet' part is about knowing what to remove from the diet and further substituting with something that does not increase inflammation. In addition, this book has shown how many functional foods can address infections commonly found in lymphoedema.

I have found that when I did try out a number of recipes - on a number of individuals with lymphoedema - that they had their own particular tastes and adapted my recipes to suit them.

It follows then that any favourite recipe can be adapted. It is not necessary to buy a bespoke recipe book. In recipes that advocate using vegetable oil, then take this out and use a stable fat such as lard or butter to sauté, for example.

If you do not generally add red wine to dishes perhaps you could consider adding a splash now and again or adding a tablespoon of tomato puree to gravy.

I add tins of tomato soup to fruit cakes as it is a 5-LO inhibitor. You cannot taste the tomato soup but it imparts a wonderful moistness to the cake which you just cannot beat.

Whenever someone has a chronic condition then they need to take control and self-manage as much as possible. One of the ways of doing this is to take responsibility for their nutritional intake and adapt their diet as they go along.

This is no different from what many other people have to do when they have a chronic condition. For example, those with high blood pressure are advised to cut down on salt. Diabetics are expected to rein in simple carbohydrates. Those who are iron deficient are advised to eat more red meat and foods containing vitamin C; vitamin C is required for iron to be absorbed by the body. All the above conditions need bespoke diets to respond to the underlying cause responsible for their symptoms. Lymphoedema is no different in this respect.

Anyway, here are a few recipes to give you a few ideas on how to adapt your diet or include foods which will help prevent the progression of lymphoedema. It may seem difficult at first especially if food preparation is not your thing but generally, after a couple of weeks, adapting meals becomes second nature.

Mixed salad

Salad items of your choice

Salad dressing made with olive oil

Wholemeal bread spread with pure almond or macadamia nut butter.

Red wine (also contains 5-LO inhibitor)

Sample meals

Tomato Soup

Ingredients

One litre of tomato juice

Two tablespoons of tomato puree

Two onions finely chopped and sautéed in butter

Teaspoon of dried basil

Bunch of fresh basil for decoration

Soured cream, small pot or you can use yogurt – please do not use fat free products or you will remove the beneficial properties of lactoferrin

Black pepper

Squeeze of lemon juice to taste

Teaspoon of sugar or sugar substitute to balance the flavours

Method

Place all the ingredients apart from the soured cream, lemon juice and fresh basil into a slow cooker.

Cook on low for 3-4 hours.

Serve with a squeeze of lemon juice, the soured cream stirred in and decorated with fresh basil.

This is a firm favourite in our family. The tomato helps suppress 5-LO and thus the inflammatory pathways involved in the development of lymphoedema. Basil is also an inhibitor and many of the other ingredients actively reduce inflammation.

It is so easy to make too. I can't be bothered with peeling and chopping onions. They are to be found in the supermarket freezing compartment already bagged up and just ready for pouring out for whatever dish is being prepared. They seem to work out cheaper, too. Of course, you can adapt these recipes to your taste. I sometimes add a little chilli to spice it up but my husband is not so keen and so I sometimes leave it out. The squeeze of lemon helps to balance the flavours out. If you don't have a lemon to hand, then add half a teaspoon of vinegar instead.

I swirl the soured cream or yogurt in the soup once the soup is in the bowl and throw chopped basil over. It looks, and tastes, delicious.

Beef Bourguignon

Ingredients

- 600g of grass fed steak, diced
- One large onion diced
- 2 garlic cloves, peeled and chopped
- Carrots peeled and chopped
- 350ml of red wine
- Sprigs of thyme to taste

- Beef stock
- Cooked dark green leafy vegetable to serve alongside

Method

Place all the ingredients – apart from the green leafy vegetable – into the slow cooker.

Cook on low heat for eight hours.

Cook green vegetable just prior to serving

Spoon a tablespoonful of olive oil onto the meat dish once it has been served out.

This is the dish that I generally make when I am having guests and I don't have time to make lots of separate dishes. It is so easy to throw everything into the slow cooker and know that it will be cooked to perfection when I am ready to serve it.

I generally serve it with rice. I have found the easiest way of cooking rice is to throw the desired amount in a large bowl and cover it with boiling water with a bit extra water so that there is about a quarter to half an inch of boiling water above the level of the rice.

Place in the microwave and cook for 10 minutes. I have never made a bad batch of rice using this method and I have shown many people how to cook rice this way. They are astonished that cooking rice can be so easy when they have been standing at the cooker stirring it around for ten minutes or so.

Choline rich shepherd's pie

12 oz of lamb's liver

Two chopped onions thinly sliced

Tomato puree to taste

1lb of cooked potato mashed with two egg yolks and a little butter

Method

Cook the liver lightly with the onions add the tomato puree and a little water to provide a little gravy

Place this in a food processor and mince.

Place in a dish and cover with the mashed potato.

Place in an oven at 180C until the potato is beginning to brown.

Eat straight away.

This was one of my children's favourites which I made often when money was tight. Liver is such a highly nutritious food and does not cost much. During the war and immediate post war years it was part of every family's weekly diet. I never had it served in a shepherd's pie though. This was one of my own inventions when I wanted to ring the changes in how liver was used.

I was fortunate that my three children all liked liver – it seems to be an acquired taste – but not one of them ever realised that the 'mince' was made from lamb's liver.

Choline rich mushroom roast

Ingredients

6 oz of mushrooms

One onion

Tablespoon of tomato puree

1 oz of butter

4 oz of grated cheese

4oz of breadcrumbs

2 egg yolks and one egg white

½ tsp of yeast extract

Seasoning as preferred

Some people like to add thyme and red wine to this recipe and it does impart a richer flavour as a whole.

Method

Chop mushroom and add to chopped onion and sauté gently in the butter until cooked.

Add the rest of the ingredients apart from the cheese. Mix well.

Press gently into a lined loaf tin, sprinkle with cheese and bake at 180C for 30 minutes.

Mushrooms, of course, do not just contain good amounts of choline. They also contain vitamin D and selenium - both excellent anti-inflammatory substances - and both tend to be lacking in most people's diets, as does choline.

If I was to be asked which three foods, we should be incorporating into our diets on a regular basis it would be

- Liver
- Eggs
- Mushrooms

Sadly, liver appears to have gone out of fashion. Most people do not like its strong taste but lamb's liver has a much milder flavour than beef or pork liver and this is the one I use in my shepherd's pies. I don't object to any kind of liver. I was brought up on it. We had it at least twice a week when I was a child. It was a cheap and highly nutritious meal.

The only contraindication for eating liver is for those who are pregnant. Liver contains large amounts of vitamin A and this can predispose to birth defects.

Choline rich bean stew

Ingredients

Assortment of colourful vegetables to taste

Mixed tinned beans: borlotti, butter, kidney, soya, for example.

Two tablespoons of tomato puree and seasoning to taste. Sage is good in this.

A tin of chopped tomatoes

A little butter to sauté vegetables in

One pint of vegetable stock

Apple puree

One and a half teaspoons of paprika pepper.

A little soured cream.

Method

Sauté the vegetables gently in the butter for three minutes.

Place in the slow cooker with the rest of the ingredients apart from the soured cream.

Turn slow cooker on high until the stew is beginning to simmer. Allow to simmer for 20 minutes and then turn down the slow cooker to low and cook for 6 hours until the vegetables are cooked through.

You need to keep an eye on the level of liquid, topping up as necessary. If the stew is too thin when you are about to serve it you can either add a tablespoon of cornflour mixed with a little cold water first or add some dried potato flakes.

Bean stew can be accompanied by just about anything. It goes well with rice, mashed potatoes, garlic bread, for examples, or it can just be eaten as it is. A dollop of yogurt or soured cream on the top works wonders.

Left to cool overnight, on being eaten the following day, the flavours have blended and intensified. It is worth preparing this dish a day ahead so that you can experience this increased richness of flavour.

If you think you will miss the addition of meat, then make sure you include borlotti beans in the stew. They have a meaty texture and are, by far, my favourite bean. My husband prefers butter beans.

If you have the time and patience, it is worth soaking and cooking bags of dried beans from scratch and freezing them for later use. This saves a lot of money as I find tinned beans very expensive when compared to the cost of the equivalent from dried beans.

I like adding red lentils to stews – normally a handful works well. They don't need soaking and thicken the stew wonderfully.

Turmeric 'coffee'

Place on teaspoonful of turmeric into a cup, stir in hot milk, sweeten to taste, if desired. This has a slightly bitter flavour and is not to everyone's taste.

Coffee sponge pudding with sauce

Ingredients

- Cupful of self-rising flour
- Cupful of pureed apple or two eggs (free range, if possible)
- Tablespoon of coffee diluted in a little water (or to taste)
- Two ounces of butter
- Sweetener or minimum sugar to taste (cupful of sugar maximum – the apple helps to sweeten the pudding)

Method

Mix all the ingredients together. Place in a pudding bowl and cover. Steam until cooked.

You may need to add a half teaspoon of baking powder if you prefer a light sponge. The addition of apple into the mix can make the sponge into a slightly denser one than many people are used to. In our household we do not have a preference.

Coffee sauce

Ingredients

- ¾ pint of milk
- Cornflour
- Sugar or sweetener to taste

Method

Take a little milk and mix with a heaped tablespoon of cornflour.

Heat the rest of the milk, add coffee to taste.

When it is just about to simmer add the milk/cornflour mix slowly, stirring all the time until the desired sauce consistency is reached. If it is not thick enough then just use a little more cornflour mixed with cold milk and add to the sauce.

Of course, you can adapt this recipe a little if you are wanting to add more choline rich foods into your diet. The recipe for Crème Anglaise below may be adapted for coffee sauce by adding coffee granules to the milk instead of vanilla essence.

Choline rich Crème Anglaise

I much prefer Crème Anglaise to the packet custard that is normally served with desserts nowadays. As it is made with egg yolks the choline content is high which helps with fat removal in the bloodstream as well as helping use fat as a source of fuel.

Ingredients

8fl oz of fresh cream

12fl oz of whole milk

4 oz of sugar or sugar substitute

½ to 1 tsp of vanilla essence

6 egg yolks

It is always better to source salmonella free eggs when making Crème Anglaise purely because this mixture is not boiled which would destroy any infective agents present.

Method

Place the cream, milk and sugar in a pan.

Bring to just off the boil. The mixture should never be allowed to boil. Take of the heat.

Whisk the egg yolks in a large bowl.

Add a little of the milk/cream mixture and whisk well. Then use this mixture to add to the milk and cream mix in the pan. Return to the heat and warm through until the egg yolks begin to thicken and take on a custard like appearance.

Once thickened, remove from the heat and add the vanilla essence and mix thoroughly.

This is better served immediately.

Baked egg custard

This was one of my grandad's favourites dishes and I have happy memories of our Sunday dinners with him which always included a baked egg custard for dessert. The eggs provide high levels of choline.

Ingredients

½ pint of milk

2-3 eggs

Rounded tablespoon of sugar

Nutmeg to sprinkle

Method

Whisk the first three ingredients together and pour into a baking dish. Sprinkle with nutmeg

Bake at 150C for approximately 45 minutes.

Tomato chaser

Add a tablespoon of olive oil to a small glass of tomato juice and drink immediately.

 Those with lymphoedema can find the day to day management of the condition stressful so to this end I have included my therapeutic bread. It is a basic recipe and can be adjusted quite easily so I need to add extra liquid I could use tomato juice and this goes especially well with dried fruit and the warm spices like nutmeg or cinnamon – the latter of which have anti-inflammatory properties.

Therapeutic bread for anxiety, stress and insomnia

porridge oats (you need to have enough to make a firm mix) so approx. 300g

3 ripened bananas

4 eggs

Handful of dried fruit (optional)

800mg of L-theanine

800mg powdered magnesium

200-400g of cooked beans

I tablespoon of sugar (optional)

I teaspoon of cinnamon

Method

Place bananas and eggs in your food processor and give a good whizz around

Place in a separate bowl with the dried fruit

Add the rest of the ingredients to the food processor – apart from the oats - and give another whizz around

Add this second mix to your egg/banana batter and give a good mix.

Leave for 15 minutes to allow the dried fruit to absorb some of the wet ingredients. (alternatively, you could soak them in a little tea first)

Stir in enough oats to make a firm consistency

Place in a well-greased loaf tin and bake at 180C for approximately 35-40 minutes or until skewer comes out clean.

Eat spread with butter.

This freezes very well.

Massage oil for lymphoedema

Olive oil is able to penetrate deeply into the skin and carry other substances with it. Olive oil can be used on its own as a massage oil. However, herbs such as oregano and thyme can be steeped in the olive oil for a few days beforehand as they also contain 5-LO inhibitors. The olive oil will help them penetrate deep into the layers of the skin. You could combine EPA with the olive oil.

In addition, as oregano and thyme contain phenolic compounds they are anti-inflammatory. In addition, they have antimicrobial properties. As such they are useful for those individuals who suffer repeated infections associated with lymphoedema.

Massage your oil into the skin gently. Cover with cling film and apply gentle warmth. Leave for about 20-30 minutes then remove gently using warm water and soap.

Make up any oil as you go along. Olive oil is also easily oxidised and must always be kept in a cool, dark place and used as quickly as possible.

Ketoprofen gel 2.5% (100g) – if you wish to try this - can be obtained from Weldricks.co.uk

The connection between Bestatin and vitamin C

At the end of this book it is probably help to go back to the beginning and look at how Bestatin works. You will recall that Bestatin was the new drug to address inflammatory systems now that it was considered that lymphoedema was not a plumbing problem.

We have already been introduced to the leukotriene LTB4, which is often shortened to B4. Leukotrienes are fatty molecules used for signalling and are active in allergies and inflammatory disorders. They help to regulate the immune system response which is the main function of signalling cells. They decide which immune system cells are needed in a response and direct them to sites of injury and inflammation. They are also involved in activating the immune system cell with especial action on the recruitment and activation of neutrophils, the kamikaze cells which hone into sites of infection, drop their toxins on the infective agent and die in the process.

Vitamin C is required in the activation of neutrophils; it is used up rapidly at times of infection so increased vitamin C is necessary. The recommendations for a respiratory infection when it is first noted to be coming on is 3g (3000mg) daily in divided doses for 3 days then 1g (1000mg) daily after that.

Neutrophils also infiltrate tissue if there is cellulitis.

 Vitamin C is also a natural B4 inhibitor so it has the same function as Bestatin but is easier to source. However, therapeutic dosages are far higher than the ineffective and measly recommended daily intake of 75mg for adult females and 90mg for adult males.

Vitamin C is easily destroyed in sunlight and heat. Cooking fruit or vegetables destroys up to 95% of the vitamin C. Much of the vitamin C will be lost during transport whether that is having travelled half way around the world or from the nearest farm.

Given today's lifestyles, the only real way to take in therapeutic levels of vitamin C is via supplementation.   The original miniscule recommended daily intakes were the very minimum set to avoid scurvy. However, for overall health, much higher amounts are needed especially in cases of infection, injury or illness. Any condition ending in 'it is' or 'oedema' will also benefit.

Vitamin C suffers from the 'familiarity breeds contempt' syndrome. It is much talked of but only with limited insight of and knowledge of its potential use in many conditions, including lymphoedema.

Prescription and over the counter medications tend to come with a huge range of negative side effects. Vitamin C, as a vital nutrient, comes without those side effects that often require the prescribing of further medications to overcome them.

The realisation that lymphoedema is an inflammatory condition instead of a 'plumbing problem' opens the way for effective natural treatments with vitamin C being the top notch vitamin in this respect.

Vitamin C works quickly too with some improvement seen within 3 days although full effect may take 3 months.

It beats the indignities of compression sleeves and other treatments which are limited and, at best, uncomfortable.

Natural medicine at its best.

One charity that has been supported through the sale of these books

A percentage of the royalties from the sale of these books are allocated for charitable purposes. One such charity that has benefitted is:

The Exodus Project

Exodus has been impacting the lives of children and young people in less advantaged communities for 20 years. Through a unique model of working, we build trusting relationships that create firm foundations for growing aspirations and regenerating communities. We target the most disadvantaged communities, trying to get kids to make the right choices for their lives.

We have learned that none of this will be achieved without long term commitment to the children and their families in these communities. Superficial remedies to deep rooted problems will only have short term impact. We are regarded as friends and not workers in the areas where we work. Our work is long established and our reputation for consistency and commitment is unquestioned. So what do we do?

We run mid-week activity clubs in the heart of the less advantaged communities of Barnsley. We bus in equipment and volunteers, to join local people in delivering exciting and fast moving activity programmes for the local kids. The programmes are great fun, as well as educational. We do dance, drama, craft, music, sports and games to entertain and energise. We also talk to the kids about the issues going on in their communities. So, if the local allotments have been broken into, or kids have been playing football on the bowling green again, we can discuss anti-social behaviour and attitudes with examples that the local young people identify with.

As well as activity clubs and home visits we take the kids away on activity weekends. We have our own activity centre, known as Jenny's Field, which we use for these weekend retreats. Jenny's Field is a home from home and a place of refuge and encouragement for so many children and young people.

The final aspect of our work might generally be termed "community partnerships". We don't want to work in isolation and we partner with parents and carers, local residents' associations, the police, housing authorities, schools and others to ensure a coordinated approach to issues on the estates.

Perhaps the most rewarding aspect of our work is the development of junior volunteers. Many of the young people who come through the activity clubs structure continue their involvement with us as leaders in the clubs where they were once members. Over the years we have nurtured hundreds of young people, sustaining relationships with them throughout their turbulent teenage years. Joe says it best:

"I very quickly fell into the family of Exodus. At such a young age nothing in my life was certain, but I knew that I belonged here. I've gone from a gobby

little kid, who used to spend hours in a porch, to a not much bigger adult with a remarkable story to tell, of how God has guided and supported me and lead me down the right path, when it would have been so easy to stray."

Facebook: TheExodusProjectBarnsley

www. exodusproject.org.uk

Thank you for your support